Ayurvedic Diet for Weight Loss

Practical Diet Recommended in Ayurveda Health System for Weight Loss and Optimum Health

Anand Gupta

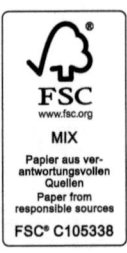

Bibliografische Information der Deutschen Nationalbibliothek:

Die Deutsche Nationalbibliothek verzeichnet diese Publikation in der Deutschen Nationalbibliografie; detaillierte bibliografische Daten sind im Internet über http://dnb.dnb.de abrufbar.

Herstellung und Verlag: BoD –
Books on Demand, Norderstedt

ISBN: 978-3-7526-1144-1

Introduction

By using this book, you accept this disclaimer in full.

No advice

The book contains information. The information is not advice and should not be treated as such.

No representations or warranties

To the maximum extent permitted by applicable law and subject to section below, we exclude all representations, warranties, undertakings and guarantees relating to the book.

Without prejudice to the generality of the foregoing paragraph, we do not represent, warrant, undertake or guarantee:

- that the information in the book is correct, accurate, complete or non-misleading.

- that the use of the guidance in the book will lead to any particular outcome or result.

Limitations and exclusions of liability

The limitations and exclusions of liability set out in this section and elsewhere in this disclaimer: are subject to section 6 below; and govern all liabilities arising under the disclaimer or in relation to the book, including liabilities arising in contract, in tort (including negligence) and for breach of statutory duty.

We will not be liable to you in respect of any losses arising out of any event or events beyond our reasonable control.

We will not be liable to you in respect of any business losses, including without limitation loss of or damage to profits, income, revenue, use, production, anticipated savings, business, contracts, commercial opportunities or goodwill.

We will not be liable to you in respect of any loss or corruption of any data, database or software.

We will not be liable to you in respect of any special, indirect or consequential loss or damage.

Exceptions

Nothing in this disclaimer shall: limit or exclude our liability for death or personal injury resulting from negligence; limit or exclude our liability for fraud or fraudulent misrepresentation; limit any of our liabilities in any way that is not permitted under applicable law; or exclude any of our liabilities that may not be excluded under applicable law.

Severability

If a section of this disclaimer is determined by any court or other competent authority to be unlawful and/or unenforceable, the other sections of this disclaimer continue in effect.

If any unlawful and/or unenforceable section would be lawful or enforceable if part of it were deleted, that part will be deemed to be deleted, and the rest of the section will continue in effect.

Law and jurisdiction

This disclaimer will be governed by and construed in accordance with Swiss law, and any disputes relating to this disclaimer will be subject to the exclusive jurisdiction of the courts of Switzerland.

Contents

Contents   **9**

Introduction   **13**

Chapter 1: Ayurvedic Diet – Getting the Basics Right   **16**

    The Kapha Dosha   *17*

    The Pitta Dosha   *20*

    The Vata Dosha   *22*

Chapter 2: Journey of a Thousand Miles – Getting Started   **25**

    Clear your food cabinets and make way for fresh foods *26*

    Eat patiently   *27*

    Know what benefits you the most   *28*

    Understand your Body   *29*

    Take a Dosha Test   *30*

    Start fine-tuning your diet   *30*

    Take your time   *31*

Chapter 3: Some Rules of the Game   **32**

    Eat when hungry   *33*

Eat patiently and comfortably   **33**

Don't eat for the heck of it   **34**

Eat warm and freshly cooked meals only   **34**

Don't eat dry foods   **34**

Be careful about the food combinations   **35**

Eat consciously   **35**

Eat your food slowly   **36**

Eat at the same time everyday   **36**

The Importance of Six Tastes in Ayurvedic Diet   **37**

Sweet   39

Sour   40

Salty   40

Pungent   41

Bitter   41

Astringent   42

Chapter 4: Tips to lose weight from Ayurvedic Diet   **44**

What, When & How of Ayurveda eating   **45**

What to eat   45

When to eat   46

How to eat   47

Conclusion   **53**

Introduction

"You are what you eat". This saying is true to the last letter and you probably heard this one before too. These words mean not only at the physical but also at psychological level. Obesity is a disease and for some reason, becoming a social taboo too. Large body is a problem not because of its appearance but because of all the health implications it subjects itself to. You can fight obesity and do so with minimal effort if you change what you eat.

Eating healthy is not a stop gap solution to obesity problem. It is a lifestyle change and a paradigm shift that you need to not only lose weight but to also maintain it.

Ayurveda is an ancient practice of medicine that teaches people to stay grounded and stay closer to earth. Ayurvedic Diet is all about eating whole foods and fresh produce. To unleash true benefits of fresh vegetables and fruits, they must be free from all the pesticides and other harmful chemicals that eat into its nutritional content.

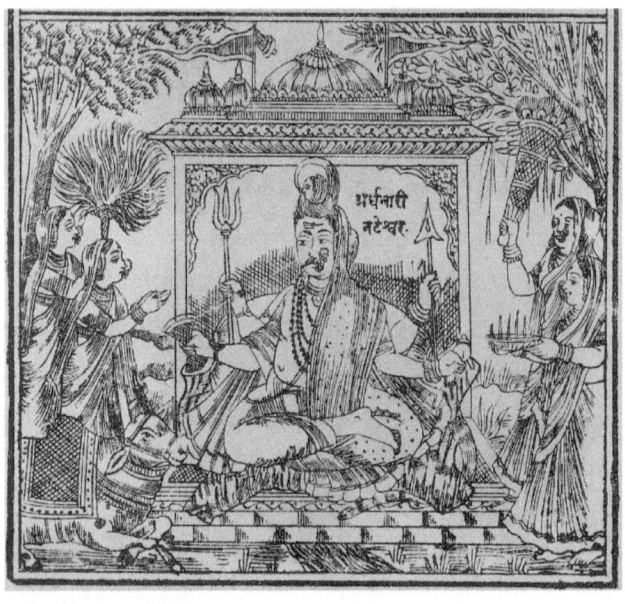

This eBook is your one stop guide to know the why's and how's of Ayurvedic dieting. I will walk you through the basics, how it helps you and how you can incorporate it into your current lifestyle. I will tell you how the eating habits that you hold so dear is killing you softly! Read this book and be amazed at all the powerful advantages of this age old practice that made its way into the modern debilitating ways by popular demand.

Chapter 1:
Ayurvedic Diet – Getting the Basics Right

Ayurveda is something that we are all briefly acquainted with, if not fully. This ancient medical system of India is an assured and fastest ways to health. This diet, unlike others, does not follow a complex rule book of do's and don'ts. It is direct, simple and unique to your body type which makes it all the more effective. When the quest is for healthy body, the guess work is best left out of the equation. The best thing about following Ayurvedic diet is that it has benefits trickling all the way down to your emotional and mental well-being too. Approaching health from a holistic viewpoint makes you feel more balanced, happy and fit and that too naturally. Ayurveda is perhaps one of those times when ancient practices trumped modernity in terms of long lasting health solutions.

To apply ayurvedic diet into your life effectively, you first need to understand your body type as defined by Ayurveda. There are three body types or dosha - Vata, Pitta and Kapha. Each of these doshas has characteristics unique to its type. While there are many ways to determine your body type, the most accurate one can be suggested by an Ayurvedic doctor.

It is common for people to associate with at least two doshas at the same time. However, one dosha is always dominant. Here I will discuss the body types briefly so that if and when you visit a professional, you know what they are talking about.

The Kapha Dosha

This dosha is attributed to the largest body type that is physically wide in hips and shoulders, good stamina and thick hair. This body type is slow in learning but have great ability to memorize. They are emotionally stable, reliable, and very trustworthy people. They are the ones that hold any relationship together by being its anchor.

People belonging to this category have an inherent misbalance in their bodies that leads to sinus congestion and poor digestion which subsequently leads to obesity. This congestion by kapha individuals can be treated by garlic supplements or diet rich in garlic. They can also go for dry body massage to stimulate the blood circulation. Dry body massage, also known as aarshana, is a specialized technique performed by raw silk gloves or can also be done by using loofah. Dry massage is the most natural way to shed water weight and also for cutting cellulite.

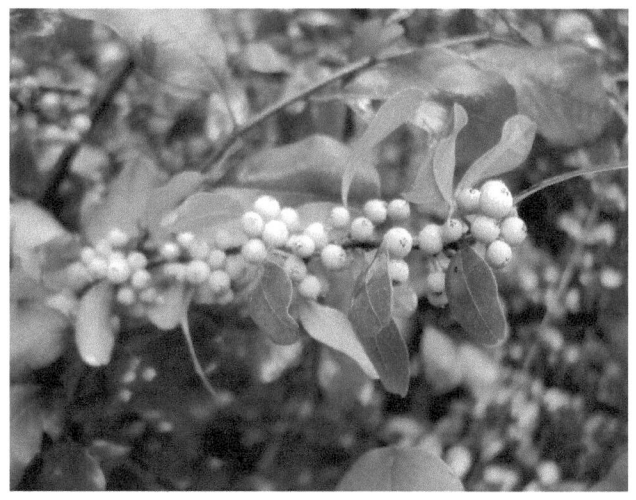

Guggul – Plant By Vinayaraj (Own work) [CC BY-SA 3.0 (http://creativecommons.org/licenses/by-sa/3.0)], via Wikimedia Commons

The metabolism can be enhanced by taking recommended herbal supplements like guggul, a plant close to myrrh. Apart from taking supplements, the kapha individuals must also exercise regularly to keep their body in perfect balance.

The dietary restrictions for these people include fat, oils, salt and sweets because of their slow-moving digestion. They should eat lots of vegetables, foods rich in fibres, cook with lots of spices and consume only fresh foods.

The Pitta Dosha

These are the medium build people that are naturally blessed with good muscle tone. They have an inherent tendency to feel warm and also suffer from premature greying of hair and even balding. They also have natural redness of complexion and envious energy levels. Because of their strong digestive system, they are able to eat just about anything. These are the people that are mentally strong, ambitious and very focused in their goals. Emotionally, these people are driven by passion and settle for nothing less than perfection.

This body type when out of balance can be gripped by excessive anger, suffer from inflammatory problems like rashes or headaches and also sometimes face digestive problems like acid reflux, ulcers etc. Because of their workaholic nature, they can feel burnt out. Pitta people can treat their inflammation problem by massaging with coconut oil to the scalp and feet before taking a shower. For preventing digestive issues, they can take half a cup of pomegranate juice with Aloe Vera juice every morning on empty stomach. For shaking off that excess stress of work, they can eat a teaspoon full of rose petal jam, alone or with a toast.

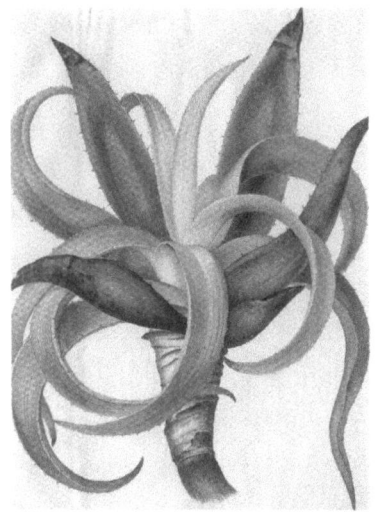

By Hans-Simon Holtzbecker (scanned from book) [Public domain], via Wikimedia Commons

Diet for pitta people should always be devoid of coffee, alcohol, spices, vinegar as well as foods with high acidic content like tomatoes. They can feast on melons and juicy fruits and also consume lots of cooling veggies like cucumber, lettuce and kale in their diets.

The Vata Dosha

This one is the most slender body type and they are the ones with skinny bodies and bony structures. They have a hard time gaining weight, are mostly cold, have dry skin and very little muscle tone. They are quick learners but have poor memories. These people are highly creative and enjoy change. Emotionally, vata types are enthusiastic and can easily become anxious.

When their body's balance is awry, Vata individuals can face poor digestion, constipation and bloating. Because of dry nasal patches, they are likely to catch cold more frequently in winters. They are easily tired and suffer from sleeplessness. People with Vata attributes should consume Triphala, an herbal supplement which is highly beneficial for people in this category. They can prevent colds due to dry nasal passage by using 1-2 sprays each morning and can fight off insomnia by following a strict daily routine. Eating, sleeping and waking up at the same to time can have many benefits on health of these people. Before bedtime, they can drink warm spiced milk.

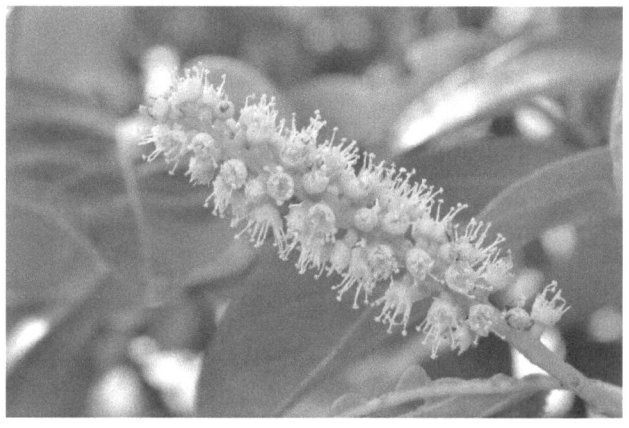

Dietary recommendations for these types of people include avoidance of carbonated drinks, dry foods and cold vegetables. They should eat well cooked meals that are soupy in nature. They can also eat cooked cereals, nuts and hot milk. They must also consume clarified butter to remove the dryness from within.

By now you should be convinced that each body type has a specific dietary requirement because of its natural formation. The only way one can truly benefit from food is when you eat what your body really needs or lacks. Once your body type is identified, your next step is to determine how to get started which brings us to our next section!

Chapter 2:
Journey of a Thousand Miles – Getting Started

Ayurveda is 5000 years old practice, tried and tested and well acclaimed Indian medical system that is gaining prominence in the Western world because of poor standards of eating. However, due to lack of adequate knowledge, some people follow it as a fad and then get disappointed when they do not see results.

Although I mentioned before, I would like to reiterate the fact that Ayurvedic Diet is not a cult following but something one does regularly with complete discipline. It is a process of a lifetime and must continue for every single day of your life. This holistic system of well-being is directed towards not only living well but also feeling well. In order to be one with yourself, you need to unite with your surroundings first and this is what Ayurvedic Dieting is all about.

According to this diet, the most important thing is to restore balance in your life though food first and then other things. Crash diets, that are so popular in the West, are so harmful that they can have implications for life if done wrong.

Ayurvedic diet does not tell you to go hungry or starve. In fact, it tells you to eat and eat well so that your body can cope with all the challenges that you face in your everyday lives.

Wondering how to get started on your Ayurvedic diet journey? Take these small yet firm steps, one at a time.

Clear your food cabinets and make way for fresh foods

Is it normal for you to be rushing through the day and shopping for groceries in a jiffy? If that is the case for you then perhaps your food cabinets are stuffed with frozen foods, quick meals and fried or fermented foods. To start on ayurvedic eating regime, the first step is to remove all these items from your food cabinet and re-place them with meals that can be freshly cooked using organic ingredients.

Eat patiently

When you are eating, try to enjoy your meals so that they are more satisfying and filling. Rushing through meals often leave you feeling dissatis-fied even when your hunger is satiated. Food has such an important part to play on your health that there is an absolutely urgent need to make it a top priority in your busy schedule. Restful breaks for meals are not just the best way to enjoy food but can also give you an en-ergy boost while making you productive soon after. Eat more consciously and with least amount of disturbance. It is also important to eat as per what your body needs most. If you are suffering from obesity then the last thing you want is to stock up on fats but you also don't want to lose the energy to perform your daily tasks. Hence, you should become the food you eat, healthy and balanced.

Know what benefits you the most

Understanding the principles of "Gunas" will help you match the food to your body type more easily. To gain the maximum benefit, it is better to know what foods are your best friends and in what way.

- "Sattvic" foods are easy to digest, organic and wholesome freshly made meals that stimulates the body and keeps your mind sharp and focused. You should eat these the most.

- "Rajasic" foods are chillies, alcohol, meat, eggs and frozen/canned foods. These foods increase stamina and are required to carry out your daily tasks but you must only consume these in moderation.

- "Tamasic" foods are leftovers from last night or mushrooms, onions and frozen/fermented foods. They need a lot of energy to digest and make us feel lethargic. They are not particularly bad foods but since we get these a lot these days, we must cut back on its intake.

Understand your Body

A professional insight from an Ayurvedic practitioner at this stage will be a good idea to learn about your body's imbalances. If you don't have a reliable doctor in your vicinity then closely observe your body to learn as much as you can.

Take a Dosha Test

You can also take a self-test to determine which dosha is prominent in your case. This will help you in building a food strategy more effectively once you know what your body requires. This is a good practice and by finding the missing pieces of what your body needs, the lifestyle change transition will become seamless.

Start fine-tuning your diet

By now you have reached a point where you are suitably aware about your body and ayurveda in general. If you feel energetic and excited to take on the challenge that lies ahead of you then you can start by fine-tuning your meals as per the knowledge that you have gained so far. It means that you can now start stocking up your food cabinets with foods that are aligned to your doshas and cook foods that are suitable for your body type. You can include those foods more that are especially good for you.

Take your time

Don't become frantic with dieting and lose steam in a few days. Let it be a slow and gradual process that you eventually incorporate in your lifestyle as a habit. Ayurveda is not about excelling at anything, be it diet or lifestyle. It is about finding harmony in your environment. Rather than marking your drawers with good and bad foods, progressively eliminate them from your eating schedule and keep them out for good.

When we are dieting, especially for weight loss, the pressure of results is so intense that we often get lost in the details and forget about the big picture. The big picture of Ayurvedic Dieting is to be healthy by eating wholesome, natural foods and what follows naturally is a weight loss that is long lasting without sucking the life out of you.

Chapter 3:
Some Rules of the Game

Knowledge these days is so readily available that one often feels overwhelmed with all the details and rules. But what I bring to you is a set of basic principles when it comes to improving digestion and is closely aligned with Ayurvedic diet values. Follow these 9 guidelines to the rote for effective ayurvedic eating.

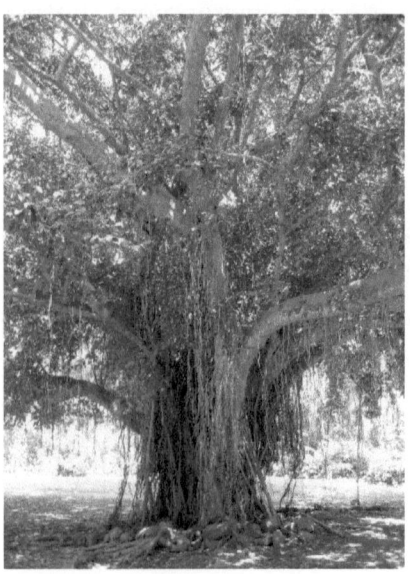

Eat when hungry

The best time to eat is when you are famished and the last meal has been digested completely. As in really hungry -- that is to say, when your previous meal has been completely digested. Sometimes dehydration seems like hunger so when you are confused between the two, just have a glass or two of water. If it quells your hunger then you have your answer!

Eat patiently and comfortably

Don't rush through your meals. Instead, sit down and avoid distractions like TV, books, phones etc. Concentrate on the food that you are eating and relish every bite.

Don't eat for the heck of it

Every single one of us is different in terms of potion size need, stomach size and metabolism rate. This is why you should only to a point where your hunger feels satiated. Listen to your body and understand the signals when your stomach is full.

Eat warm and freshly cooked meals only

Avoid eating anything straight from the fridge if you want to preserve the digestive system. Hot meals work wonders for your metabolism and helps in quick digestion of the food.

Don't eat dry foods

Juicy or slightly oily foods are necessary for your body as some nutrients are oil soluble only. They will not be absorbed by your body if you only eat dry foods. You can eat healthy oils like olive oil or coconut oil that are rich in good fat and are healthy for your body.

Be careful about the food combinations

Did you know that some of your favourite food pairings can actually be making you sick? Food needs to be paired carefully so that they can together do the good that they are supposed. Bad food combinations can actually make your stomach upset and lead to bigger problems later. Some common food combinations that you can avoid on Ayurvedic Diet is banana and milk, fruit and yogurt, lemon dressing on cucumber and tomato salad etc.

Eat consciously

Appreciate the food that you eat and engage all the 5 senses when you eat. Once you are fully engaged with the food, you will see how fulfilling each meal becomes.

Eat your food slowly

Chewing is the first step to digest your food. Eat slowly, carefully breaking down your food and enjoying every bite of it.

Eat at the same time everyday

Nature works best when your body follows routine. So eat every day at the same time for your own good.

The Importance of Six Tastes in Ayurvedic Diet

The best thing about following Ayurvedic diet is that it recognizes the importance of taste in food which makes it easier to stick to the dieting plan. It uses taste to its advantage and gives you the results that you are yearning for.

There are six tastes that our body needs and must definitely form a part of our food to make us feel satisfied at the end of your meals. The six tastes are:

Sweet – sugar, honey, rice, pasta, milk, etc

Salty – salt, any salty food

Sour – lemons, hard cheese, yogurt, vinegar, etc.

Bitter – leafy greens, turmeric, lettuce, etc.

Pungent – chili peppers, cayenne, ginger, any hot spice

Astringent –beans, pomegranate, lentils, etc.

Cravings are resulted because one of the tastes from these six has been left unsatisfied. Don't be one of those people who omit the bitter and astringent taste from their foods. Did you know that eating something astringent or bitter after your meal can actually reduce your longing for sweets?

Adding all these tastes to your ayurvedic diet can improve your health significantly and also help in incorporating ayurvedic way of life into your lifestyle.

Every single taste is composed of two elements such as - sweet taste is made up of earth and water, sour is fire and water, salty is earth and fire, bitter is air and ether, astringent is air and earth and pungent is fire and air. These elements are rich in their respective attributes or gunas that can greatly influence your mental and physical condition.

These tastes are used by Ayurvedic Diet which follows a medicine-science approach pro-moting holistic well-being and good health.

Here I have listed all the tastes in order of their digestion. After you read this, I assure you that you will never eat your dessert after your meals!

Sweet

Sweet taste is made of water and earth elements and is associated with kapha qualities. It is inherently cold and heavy as well as highly nourishing. In fact it the most nourishing taste of all the tastes. Sweet food nurtures our tissue and blood plasma and cultivates our contact with the body so that we can stay grounded and enjoy life more. It is also said that sweet food enhances fertility but too much sweet food can make the body feel lethargic. Sweet foods include cereals, pumpkin and dates.

Sour

This taste is composed of water and fire. Sour taste foods must be eaten in moderation as too much or too less can lead to ill effects on the body. For instance, too much sour taste can result in infections and make you feel aggressive. However, in the right quantities, it awakens the mind and alerts the thoughts as well as emotions to become clear. It is also good at enhancing digestion but too much can weaken the fertility of the body. Some sour foods include lemon, tamarind, wine etc.

Salty

Salty taste is made up of earth and fire. Salt can only be found in minerals and not in plants. Adequate salt taste can solidify the body and adds taste to the foods. Everything tastes better when you add a pinch of salt and it helps in digesting foods more easily. However, too much salt in foods can be very harmful. Some examples of salty foods include Himalayan salt, rock salt, sea salt etc.

Pungent

This taste consists of fire and air elements. Pungent foods help in stimulating the digestion. It is also very good for clearing our thinking thus helping us in understanding complex matters effortlessly. On the other hand, too much pungent food can also lead to infections and haemorrhages. Pungent foods include spices, pepper and ginger.

Bitter

Bitter taste is composed of ether and air. This type of food is especially suitable for people with Kapha body type and is very helpful in increasing strength. Because of its cooling properties, bitter taste foods are also purifying in nature that helps in removing waste products from our body. Bitter foods are especially beneficial in purifying the mind. It rids the mind of stifling emotions and obsessions. However, too much of it can make you bitter. Examples of bitter foods are green tea and veggies.

Astringent

This taste comprises of air and earth. All those people that fall in the kapha body type category can benefit from this taste. Astringent food is ideal at defeating the problem of limpness and weakness. This taste is also good at purifying and strengthening your brain. This food is especially useful in creating the balance that the bodies normally lack. However, too much of it can make you nihilistic. Green vegetables and curcuma are the examples of astringent foods.

The knowledge about these tastes is very help-ful when your doshas are not in balance. When eaten in right proportion and with alignment of your doshas, they can do wonders in restoring the lost balance. If your body is in a healthy state, you can include these in your diet and bring all the elements of nature in your food.

Chapter 4:
Tips to lose weight from Ayurvedic Diet

We sadly live in a society that demonizes large bodies not for its health implications but because it does not meet the socially acceptable standards of beauty. This kind of mindset is making it hard for people to stay focused and make them feel stressed. Did you know that stress is one of the biggest reasons for weight increase?

Ayurvedic diet comes for rescue but to what end? It is important for all the people to realize that is ancient old practice must be incorporated for life and not only until you get the much coveted beach body!

Here is how you can include Ayurvedic food into your eating schedule.

What, When & How of Ayurveda eating

The three most important aspect of ayurvedic diet lies in what, when and how you eat. Let's discuss each of these aspects individually.

What to eat

The best foods to eat are the ones that are harvested as per the season they grew in. Nature is very forthcoming when it comes to our bodily needs. For instance, you must eat high fat diet in winter to keep you warm and active while eating low fat and mucous reducing foods like sprouts, berries, root veggies etc in spring season to treat seasonal allergies. Since all these food burn fat and toxins, they are the ideal spring foods.

For summers, since the months are hot, the nature harvests cool fruits that help us from getting dried out or overheated.

To put it simply, there is no such thing as bad foods. When you are eating ayurvedic, you need to focus on the foods that you should eat more of in their respective seasons.

If you have learnt to eat six meals a day, you must unlearn that right now. Six-meal diet is not a way of life but a medicine to treat low blood sugar problem. The right thing to do will be to not allow your blood sugar levels to dip dangerously low.

To start with healthy weight loss process, start by eating three proper meals and no snacks in between. This will soon train your body to make the blood sugar last from one meal to another. Meanwhile, your body will burn fat for fuel in between meals. However, if you snack during this time, your body doesn't feel the need to burn its fat storage.

The best time to eat your biggest meal is during the first half of the day, between 10 AM and 2 PM since the digestion is the strongest during this time. By sticking to this routine, your body

will be able to get rid of its midday sugar cravings in a matter of 2 weeks.

How to eat

Eat each meal when you are seated comfortably
and minus all the distractions. Enjoy your well
prepared meals in a relaxed social setting. This is
important to create harmony between mind and
body when we are eating. Your digestion works
best when it is relaxed. As a result, your mind is
as nourished as your body and you can experi-
ence the full benefits of balanced meals.

Ayurvedic Diet is a great way to lose weight in a
healthy manner that does not only cure obesity
but also promotes habit of perpetual healthy living. Ayurveda was developed thousands of
years ago in India and is considered as an exten-
sion of Yoga. The thing that equates both these
techniques is that they focus on restoring balance in mind, body and soul, cultivating healthy

habits and following the guidelines that are in sync with nature's rhythms as well as seasons.

You can start following these tips that will help lose weight organically and guide you to a life of healthy and holistic weight loss without using anything that does not come directly from nature.

1. The best way to stimulate your bowels in the morning is to have a large glass of warm water with lemon the first thing when you wake up. Drink this on empty stomach and give yourself a fresh start of the day.

2. Exercise at least 45-60 minutes each day and long enough to break a sweat. If you follow this early morning practice every day, you can easily lose weight without breaking your back. Choose a form of exercise that you can do everyday for the rest of your life and follow it religiously.

3. Practice yoga/meditation for at least 10-15 minutes every day so that you can

make your mind and body feel relaxed and take on day's challenges with renewed fervour. This is the best way to alleviate stress and earn more focus for your day's important activities. Stress is one of the main reasons for weight gain that can be easily trumped by relaxing your mind with yoga and meditation techniques.

4. Eat three full meals and avoid snacking in between. Your body forgets its fat burning function when it is constantly fed with food. Start with a moderate meal in the morning between 7.30-9.00 AM. Your biggest meal should be between lunch time of 12.00-2.00 PM and the smallest meal should be dinner between 5.30 PM and 8.00 PM.

5. Align your eating habits with the time of the day and season. Summers get long and hot and in that season, the fruits and vegetables are naturally rich in carbohydrates to keep the body cool as well as

active. However, in winter months what you see a lot of root vegetables, nuts, fruits and seeds, cheese, heavy meats, stored grains etc. All these foods are inherently warm thus keeping us balmy in winter chills. When the season is damp in spring, nature grows lots of green leafy vegetables and berries as well as sprouts to cleanse our bodies from days of heavy winter eating. When we eat naturally and feast on seasonal produce, our bodies accumulate all the necessary nutrients.

6. Do not forget to add all the six tastes of ayurveda food in your diet – sweet, sour, bitter, salty, pungent and astringent. All these elements of taste together work in harmony to restore balance in our bodies from within. Since we consume too much sweet, salt and sour taste in diets these days, it quickly became major cause of weight gain. However, other foods like bitter leafy greens, pungent spicy peppers and astringent

pomegranate seeds in the food will off-set the ill effects of excess of salt, sour and sweet.

7.   After every meal, it is always better to move a little. When you walk after dinner, it does wonders in improving digestion. Do the same after lunch as well and walk for at least 10-20 minutes at a moderate pace. You can further improve digestion if you can lie on your left side after walking for 10 minutes.

8.   You can create a major hormone balance in your body if you can manage to sleep at dusk and rise at dawn each morning. Tapping into your circadian rhythms is the best thing you can do to your body in terms of natural balances. Back in the day, our ancestors had nothing to keep them awake at night so they naturally slowed down as the sun went down. However, today our bright phone screens or that of our laptops keep our brains awake and prevent us from

sleeping fitfully at night. Sleeping for a minimum of 7 hours and maximum of 9 hours each day helps our bodies reset for next day. This also maintains healthy cortisol levels that cause weight gain.

These tips are geared towards natural weight loss and also have profound impact on your lives. Following these steps in conjunction with balanced ayurvedic diet will have the most impactful and stress free weight loss. You can take one step at a time approach or incorporate this plan fully into your routine. The trick is to stay as close to nature as possible if you want to lose your weight and not your mind.

Conclusion

Ayurvedic dieting is all about eating and eating well. Weight gain is not because of how much we eat it is about how much of what we eat. This is exactly the problem that ayurvedic diet addresses through its core tenets.

Through this eBook I have tried to build a relation between nature and food through the principles of Ayurveda that not only helps in healthy weight loss but also focuses on holistic well-being.

I have used tips and basic knowledge to educate you about this diet form so that you can make an informed choice equipped with all the core information that forms the basis of Ayurvedic dieting.